Essential Oil Journal Recipe notebook

This Journal Belongs To:

_____

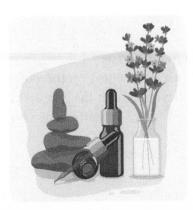

First Printing, 2019

ISBN 9781798291573

Index

Recipe	Page

Index

Recipe	Page

Index

Recipe   Page

Recipe _____

Ingredients:

_____
_____
_____
_____
_____
_____
_____
_____
_____

Directions:

_____
_____
_____
_____
_____
_____
_____

Uses:

_____
_____

Recipe _____

Ingredients:

_____

_____

_____

_____

_____

_____

_____

_____

_____

_____

Directions:

_____

_____

_____

_____

_____

_____

Uses:

_____

_____

Recipe _____

Ingredients:

Directions:

Uses:

8

Recipe _____

Ingredients:

_____

_____

_____

_____

_____

_____

_____

_____

_____

_____

Directions:

_____

_____

_____

_____

_____

_____

Uses:

_____

_____

Recipe _____

Ingredients: _____

_____

_____

_____

_____

_____

_____

_____

_____

Directions: _____

_____

_____

_____

_____

_____

Uses: _____

_____

10

Recipe _____

Ingredients:

_____

_____

_____

_____

_____

_____

_____

_____

_____

Directions:

_____

_____

_____

_____

_____

_____

_____

Uses:

_____

_____

Recipe _____

Ingredients:

Directions:

Uses:

Recipe _____

Ingredients: _____

_____

_____

_____

_____

_____

_____

_____

_____

_____

Directions: _____

_____

_____

_____

_____

_____

Uses: _____

_____

_____

Recipe _____

Ingredients:

Directions:

Uses:

Recipe _____

Ingredients:

_____

_____

_____

_____

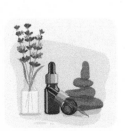

_____

_____

_____

_____

_____

Directions:

_____

_____

_____

_____

_____

_____

Uses:

_____

_____

Recipe _____

Ingredients:

Directions:

Uses:

16

Recipe _____

Ingredients: _____
_____
_____
_____
_____
_____
_____
_____
_____
_____
_____
_____

Directions: _____
_____
_____
_____
_____
_____
_____
_____
_____

Uses: _____
_____
_____
_____

Recipe _____

Ingredients:

Directions:

Uses:

18

Recipe _____

Ingredients:

_____

_____

_____

_____

_____

_____

_____

_____

_____

Directions:

_____

_____

_____

_____

_____

_____

Uses:

_____

_____

_____

Recipe _____

Ingredients:

_____

_____

_____

_____

_____

_____

_____

_____

Directions:

_____

_____

_____

_____

_____

_____

Uses:

_____

_____

Recipe _____

Ingredients:

_____

_____

_____

_____

_____

_____

_____

_____

_____

_____

Directions:

_____

_____

_____

_____

_____

Uses:

_____

_____

Recipe _____

Ingredients:

Directions:

Uses:

Recipe _____

Ingredients:

_____

_____

_____

_____

_____

_____

_____

_____

Directions:

_____

_____

_____

_____

_____

_____

Uses:

_____

_____

Recipe _____

Ingredients:
_____
_____
_____
_____

_____
_____
_____
_____

Directions:
_____
_____
_____
_____
_____

Uses:
_____
_____
_____

Recipe _____

Ingredients:

_____

_____

_____

_____

_____

_____

_____

_____

_____

Directions:

_____

_____

_____

_____

_____

_____

Uses:

_____

_____

Recipe _____

Ingredients:

Directions:

Uses:

Recipe _____

Ingredients: _____

_____
_____
_____
_____
_____
_____
_____
_____
_____
_____
_____

Directions: _____

_____
_____
_____
_____
_____
_____
_____

Uses: _____

_____
_____

Recipe _____

Ingredients:

_____

_____

_____

_____

_____

_____

_____

_____

Directions:

_____

_____

_____

_____

_____

_____

Uses:

_____

_____

Recipe _____

Ingredients:

_____

_____

_____

_____

_____

_____

_____

_____

_____

_____

_____

_____

_____

Directions:

_____

_____

_____

_____

_____

_____

_____

Uses:

_____

_____

Recipe _____

Ingredients:

Directions:

Uses:

30

Recipe _____

Ingredients:

_____

_____

_____

_____

_____

_____

_____

_____

_____

Directions:

_____

_____

_____

_____

_____

_____

Uses:

_____

_____

Recipe _____

Ingredients:

_____

_____

_____

_____

_____

_____

_____

_____

Directions:

_____

_____

_____

_____

_____

Uses:

_____

_____

_____

Recipe _____

Ingredients:
_____

_____

_____

_____

_____

_____

_____

_____

_____

Directions:
_____

_____

_____

_____

_____

Uses:
_____

_____

_____

Recipe _____

Ingredients:

Directions:

Uses:

Recipe _____

Ingredients:

_____

_____

_____

_____

_____

_____

_____

_____

_____

Directions:

_____

_____

_____

_____

_____

_____

Uses:

_____

_____

Recipe _____

Ingredients:

_____

_____

_____

_____

_____

_____

_____

Directions:

_____

_____

_____

_____

_____

Uses:

_____

_____

Recipe _____

Ingredients:

_____
_____
_____
_____
_____
_____
_____
_____
_____
_____
_____

Directions:

_____
_____
_____
_____
_____
_____
_____

Uses:

_____
_____
_____

Recipe _____

Ingredients:

Directions:

Uses:

38

Recipe _____

Ingredients:
_____

_____

_____

_____

_____

_____

_____

_____

_____

_____

Directions:
_____

_____

_____

_____

_____

_____

Uses:
_____

_____

Recipe _____

Ingredients:

_____

_____

_____

_____

_____

_____

_____

_____

Directions:

_____

_____

_____

_____

_____

_____

Uses:

_____

_____

_____

Recipe _____

Ingredients:

_____
_____
_____
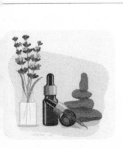
_____
_____
_____
_____
_____
_____

Directions:

_____
_____
_____
_____
_____
_____

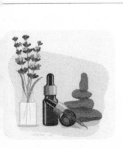

Uses:

_____
_____

Recipe _____

Ingredients:

Directions:

Uses:

42

Recipe _____

Ingredients:

_____

_____

_____

_____

_____

_____

_____

_____

_____

_____

Directions:

_____

_____

_____

_____

_____

_____

_____

Uses:

_____

_____

Recipe _____

Ingredients:

Directions:

Uses:

Recipe _____

Ingredients:

_____

_____

_____

_____

_____

_____

_____

_____

_____

_____

Directions:

_____

_____

_____

_____

_____

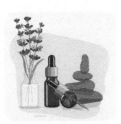

Uses:

_____

_____

_____

Recipe _____

Ingredients:

_____

_____

_____

_____

_____

_____

_____

_____

_____

Directions:

_____

_____

_____

_____

_____

_____

Uses:

_____

_____

Recipe _____

Ingredients: _____
_____
_____
_____
_____
_____
_____
_____
_____
_____
_____

Directions: _____
_____
_____
_____
_____
_____
_____

Uses: _____
_____
_____

Recipe _____

Ingredients:

Directions:

Uses:

Recipe _____

Ingredients:

_____

_____

_____

_____

_____

_____

_____

_____

_____

Directions:

_____

_____

_____

_____

_____

_____

Uses:

_____

_____

Recipe _____

Ingredients:
_____
_____
_____
_____
_____
_____
_____
_____
_____

Directions:
_____
_____
_____
_____
_____
_____

Uses:
_____
_____
_____

Recipe _____

Ingredients:

_____

_____

_____

_____

_____

_____

_____

_____

Directions:

_____

_____

_____

_____

_____

Uses:

_____

_____

_____

Recipe _____

Ingredients:
_____
_____
_____
_____
_____
_____
_____
_____

Directions:
_____
_____
_____
_____
_____

Uses:
_____
_____

Recipe _____

Ingredients:

_____

_____

_____

_____

_____

_____

_____

_____

_____

Directions:

_____

_____

_____

_____

_____

_____

Uses:

_____

_____

Recipe _____

Ingredients:

_____

_____

_____

_____

_____

_____

_____

_____

_____

Directions:

_____

_____

_____

_____

_____

_____

Uses:

_____

_____

Recipe _____

Ingredients:

_____

_____

_____

_____

_____

_____

_____

_____

_____

_____

Directions:

_____

_____

_____

_____

_____

Uses:

_____

_____

Recipe _____

Ingredients:

_____

_____

_____

_____

_____

_____

_____

_____

_____

Directions:

_____

_____

_____

_____

_____

_____

Uses:

_____

_____

Recipe _____

Ingredients:

_____

_____

_____

_____

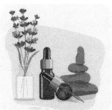

_____

_____

_____

_____

_____

_____

Directions:

_____

_____

_____

_____

_____

_____

Uses:

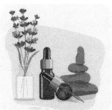

_____

_____

Recipe _____

Ingredients:

Directions:

Uses:

58

Recipe _____

Ingredients:

_____

_____

_____

_____

_____

_____

_____

_____

_____

_____

_____

Directions:

_____

_____

_____

_____

_____

_____

_____

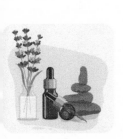

Uses:

_____

_____

Recipe _____

Ingredients:
_____
_____
_____
_____
_____
_____
_____
_____

Directions:
_____
_____
_____
_____
_____

Uses:
_____
_____
_____

Recipe _____

Ingredients:

_____

_____

_____

_____

_____

_____

_____

_____

_____

Directions:

_____

_____

_____

_____

_____

_____

Uses:

_____

_____

Recipe _____

Ingredients:

_____
_____
_____
_____
_____
_____
_____
_____
_____

Directions:

_____
_____
_____
_____
_____

Uses:

_____
_____

Recipe _____

Ingredients:

_____

_____

_____

_____

_____

_____

_____

_____

_____

Directions:

_____

_____

_____

_____

_____

Uses:

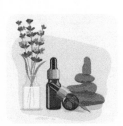

_____

_____

Recipe _____

Ingredients:

_____

_____

_____

_____

_____

_____

_____

_____

Directions:

_____

_____

_____

_____

_____

_____

Uses:

_____

_____

Recipe _____

Ingredients:

_____

_____

_____

_____

_____

_____

_____

_____

_____

_____

Directions:

_____

_____

_____

_____

_____

_____

Uses:

_____

_____

_____

Recipe _____

Ingredients:

_____

_____

_____

_____

_____

_____

_____

_____

Directions:

_____

_____

_____

_____

_____

_____

Uses:

_____

_____

Recipe _____

Ingredients:

_____

_____

_____

_____

_____

_____

_____

_____

_____

Directions:

_____

_____

_____

_____

_____

_____

Uses:

_____

_____

Recipe _____

Ingredients:
_____
_____
_____
_____
_____
_____
_____
_____
_____
_____

Directions:
_____
_____
_____
_____
_____
_____

Uses:
_____
_____

Recipe _____

Ingredients:

_____

_____

_____

_____

_____

_____

_____

_____

_____

Directions:

_____

_____

_____

_____

_____

_____

Uses:

_____

_____

Recipe _____

Ingredients:

_____

_____

_____

_____

_____

_____

_____

_____

_____

Directions:

_____

_____

_____

_____

_____

_____

Uses:

_____

_____

Recipe _____

Ingredients:

_____

_____

_____

_____

_____

_____

_____

_____

_____

_____

Directions:

_____

_____

_____

_____

_____

_____

_____

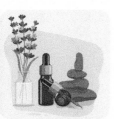

Uses:

_____

_____

_____

Recipe _____

Ingredients:

_____

_____

_____

_____

_____

_____

_____

Directions:

_____

_____

_____

_____

_____

Uses:

_____

_____

Recipe _____

Ingredients:

_____
_____
_____
_____
_____
_____
_____
_____
_____
_____
_____

Directions:

_____
_____
_____
_____
_____
_____

Uses:

_____
_____

Recipe _____

Ingredients:

_____

_____

_____

_____

_____

_____

_____

_____

Directions:

_____

_____

_____

_____

_____

Uses:

_____

_____

Recipe _____

Ingredients:

_____

_____

_____

_____

_____

_____

_____

_____

_____

Directions:

_____

_____

_____

_____

_____

Uses:

_____

_____

Recipe _____

Ingredients:
_____
_____
_____
_____
_____
_____
_____
_____
_____

Directions:
_____
_____
_____
_____
_____

Uses:
_____
_____

Recipe _____

Ingredients:

_____

_____

_____

_____

_____

_____

_____

_____

_____

Directions:

_____

_____

_____

_____

_____

Uses:

_____

_____

Recipe _____

Ingredients:

_____

_____

_____

_____

_____

_____

_____

_____

_____

Directions:

_____

_____

_____

_____

_____

_____

Uses:

_____

_____

Recipe _____

Ingredients:

_____

_____
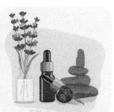
_____

_____

_____

_____

_____

_____

_____

_____

_____

Directions:

_____

_____

_____

_____

_____

_____

_____

Uses:

_____

_____

_____

Recipe _____

Ingredients:
_____
_____
_____
_____
_____
_____
_____
_____

Directions:
_____
_____
_____
_____
_____

Uses:
_____
_____

Recipe _____

Ingredients:

_____

_____

_____

_____

_____

_____

_____

_____

_____

_____

Directions:

_____

_____

_____

_____

_____

_____

Uses:

_____

_____

Recipe _____

Ingredients:

Directions:

Uses:

82

Recipe _____

Ingredients:

_____

_____

_____

_____

_____

_____

_____

_____

_____

_____

Directions:

_____

_____

_____

_____

_____

Uses:

_____

_____

_____

Recipe _____

Ingredients:

_____

_____

_____

_____

_____

_____

_____

_____

Directions:

_____

_____

_____

_____

_____

Uses:

_____

_____

Recipe _____

Ingredients:

_____

_____

_____

_____

_____

_____

_____

_____

_____

_____

Directions:

_____

_____

_____

_____

_____

Uses:

_____

_____

_____

Recipe _____

Ingredients:

Directions:

Uses:

Recipe _____

Ingredients:

_____

_____

_____

_____

_____

_____

_____

_____

Directions:

_____

_____

_____

_____

_____

Uses:

_____

_____

_____

Recipe _____

Ingredients:
_____
_____
_____
_____
_____
_____
_____
_____

Directions:
_____
_____
_____
_____
_____
_____

Uses:
_____
_____

Recipe _____

Ingredients:

_____

_____

_____

_____

_____

_____

_____

_____

_____

Directions:

_____

_____

_____

_____

_____

_____

Uses:

_____

_____

Recipe _____

Ingredients:

_____

_____

_____

_____

_____

_____

_____

_____

Directions:

_____

_____

_____

_____

_____

Uses:

_____

_____

Recipe _____

Ingredients:

_____

_____

_____

_____

_____

_____

_____

_____

_____

Directions:

_____

_____

_____

_____

_____

Uses:

_____

_____

Recipe _____

Ingredients:

_____
_____
_____
_____
_____
_____
_____
_____

Directions:

_____
_____
_____
_____
_____
_____

Uses:

_____
_____

Recipe _____

Ingredients:

_____

_____

_____

_____

_____

_____

_____

_____

Directions:

_____

_____

_____

_____

_____

Uses:

_____

_____

_____

Recipe _____

Ingredients:

_____
_____
_____
_____
_____
_____
_____
_____
_____

Directions:

_____
_____
_____
_____
_____
_____

Uses:

_____
_____

Recipe _____

Ingredients:

_____

_____

_____

_____

_____

_____

_____

_____

_____

Directions:

_____

_____

_____

_____

_____

_____

Uses:

_____

_____

Recipe _____

Ingredients:
_____
_____
_____
_____
_____
_____
_____
_____
_____

Directions:
_____
_____
_____
_____
_____
_____

Uses:
_____
_____
_____

Recipe _____

Ingredients:

_____

_____

_____

_____

_____

_____

_____

_____

_____

_____

_____

Directions:

_____

_____

_____

_____

_____

_____

_____

Uses:

_____

_____

_____

Recipe _____

Ingredients:

_____

_____

_____

_____

_____

_____

_____

_____

Directions:

_____

_____

_____

_____

_____

Uses:

_____

_____

Recipe _____

Ingredients:

_____
_____
_____
_____
_____
_____
_____
_____
_____

Directions:

_____
_____
_____
_____
_____

Uses:

_____
_____

Recipe _____

Ingredients:
_____
_____
_____
_____
_____
_____
_____
_____

Directions:
_____
_____
_____
_____
_____

Uses:
_____
_____

Recipe _____

Ingredients:

_____
_____
_____
_____
_____
_____
_____
_____
_____
_____
_____

Directions:

_____
_____
_____
_____
_____
_____

Uses:

_____
_____

Recipe _____

Ingredients:

_____

_____

_____

_____

_____

_____

_____

_____

Directions:

_____

_____

_____

_____

_____

Uses:

_____

_____

Recipe _____

Ingredients:

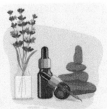

Directions:

Uses:

Recipe _____

Ingredients:

_____
_____
_____
_____
_____
_____
_____
_____

Directions:

_____
_____
_____
_____
_____
_____

Uses:

_____
_____

Recipe _____

Ingredients:

_____

_____

_____

_____

_____

_____

_____

_____

_____

Directions:

_____

_____

_____

_____

_____

_____

Uses:

_____

_____

_____

Recipe _____

Ingredients:

Directions:

Uses:

Recipe _____

Ingredients:

_____

_____

_____

_____

_____

_____

_____

_____

_____

Directions:

_____

_____

_____

_____

_____

_____

Uses:

_____

_____

_____

Recipe _____

Ingredients:
_____
_____
_____
_____
_____
_____
_____
_____
_____

Directions:
_____
_____
_____
_____
_____
_____

Uses:
_____
_____
_____

108

Recipe _____

Ingredients:

_____

_____

_____

_____

_____

_____

_____

_____

_____

Directions:

_____

_____

_____

_____

_____

_____

Uses:

_____

_____

Recipe _____

Ingredients:

_____
_____
_____
_____
_____
_____
_____
_____
_____

Directions:

_____
_____
_____
_____
_____
_____

Uses:

_____
_____

Recipe _____

Ingredients:
_____

_____

_____

_____

_____

_____

_____

_____

Directions:
_____

_____

_____

_____

_____

_____

Uses:
_____

_____

_____

Recipe _____

Ingredients:

Directions:

Uses:

Recipe _____

Ingredients:

_____

_____

_____

_____

_____

_____

_____

_____

Directions:

_____

_____

_____

_____

_____

Uses:

_____

_____

Recipe _____

Ingredients:

_____

_____

_____

_____

_____

_____

_____

_____

Directions:

_____

_____

_____

_____

_____

Uses:

_____

_____

Recipe _____

Ingredients:

_____

_____

_____

_____

_____

_____

_____

_____

_____

Directions:

_____

_____

_____

_____

_____

Uses:

_____

_____

Recipe _____

Ingredients:

_____

_____

_____

_____

_____

_____

_____

_____

_____

Directions:

_____

_____

_____

_____

_____

_____

Uses:

_____

_____

Recipe _____

Ingredients: _____

_____

_____

_____

_____

_____

_____

_____

_____

Directions: _____

_____

_____

_____

_____

_____

Uses: _____

_____

_____

Recipe _____

Ingredients:

Directions:

Uses:

118

Recipe _____

Ingredients:

_____

_____

_____

_____

_____

_____

_____

_____

_____

Directions:

_____

_____

_____

_____

_____

_____

Uses:

_____

_____

Recipe _____

Ingredients:

Directions:

Uses:

Recipe _____

Ingredients:

_____

_____

_____

_____

_____

_____

_____

_____

_____

Directions:

_____

_____

_____

_____

_____

_____

Uses:

_____

_____

Recipe _____

Ingredients:

Directions:

Uses:

Recipe _____

Ingredients:

_____

_____

_____

_____

_____

_____

_____

_____

_____

_____

_____

Directions:

_____

_____

_____

_____

_____

_____

Uses:

_____

_____